MedicalCenter.com

I0439906

The Key Facts
On Cancer Detection &
Diagnosis

The Key Facts on Cancer: Volume V

Everything You Need to Know About Cancer Detection & Diagnosis

-Usable Medical Information for the Patient-

By Patrick W. Nee

www.MedicalCenter.com

Published by:

MedicalCenter.com

96 Walter Street/ Suite 200

Boston, MA 02131, USA

Tel: 617-354-7722

www.MedicalCenter.com

manager@medicalcenter.com

The Key Facts on Cancer Series

Table of Contents

Chapter 1: Introduction

What is Cancer?

Cancer is a term used for diseases in which abnormal cells divide without control and are able to invade other tissues. Cancer cells can spread to other parts of the body through the blood and lymph systems.

Cancer is not just one disease but many diseases. There are more than 100 different types of cancer. Most cancers are named for the organ or type of cell in which they start - for example, cancer that begins in the colon is called colon cancer; cancer that begins in melanocytes of the skin is called melanoma.

Cancer types can be grouped into broader categories. The main categories of cancer include:

- *Carcinoma*- cancer that begins in the skin or in tissues that line or cover internal organs. There are a number of subtypes of carcinoma, including adenocarcinoma, basal cell carcinoma,squamous cell carcinoma, and transitional cell carcinoma.

- *Sarcoma* - cancer that begins in bone, cartilage, fat, muscle, blood vessels, or other connective or supportive tissue.

- *Leukemia* - cancer that starts in blood-forming tissue such as the bone marrow and causes large numbers of abnormal blood cells to be produced and enter the blood.

- *Lymphoma and myeloma* - cancers that begin in the cells of the immune system.

- *Central nervous system cancers* - cancers that begin in the tissues of the brain and spinal cord.

Origins of Cancer

All cancers begin in cells, the body's basic unit of life. To understand cancer, it's helpful to know what happens when normal cells become cancer cells.

The body is made up of many types of cells. These cells grow and divide in a controlled way to produce more cells as they are needed to keep the body healthy. When cells become old or damaged, they die and are replaced with new cells. However, sometimes this orderly process goes wrong. The genetic material (DNA) of a cell can become damaged or changed, producing mutations that affect normal cell growth and division. When this happens, cells do not die when they should and new cells form when the body does not need them. The extra cells may form a mass of tissue called a tumor.

Not all tumors are cancerous; tumors can be benign or malignant.

- ***Benign tumors*** aren't cancerous. They can often be removed, and, in most cases, they do not come back. Cells in benign tumors do not spread to other parts of the body.

- ***Malignant tumors*** are cancerous. Cells in these tumors can invade nearby tissues and spread to other parts of the body. The spread of cancer from one part of the body to another is called metastasis.

Some cancers do not form tumors. For example, leukemia is a cancer of the bone marrow and blood.

Cancer Statistics

A report from the nation's leading cancer organizations shows that rates of death in the United States from all cancers for men and women continued to fall between 2005 and 2009, the most recent reporting period available.

Estimated new cases and deaths from cancer in the United States in 2013:

- *New cases*: 1,660,290 (does not include nonmelanoma skin cancers)
- *Deaths*: 580,350

The risk of developing many types of cancer can be reduced by practicing healthy lifestyle habits, such as eating a healthy diet, getting regular exercise, and not smoking. Also, the sooner a cancer is found and treatment begins, the better the chances are that the treatment will be successful.

Chapter 2: Cancer Staging

- Staging describes the extent or severity of a person's cancer. Knowing the stage of disease helps the doctor plan treatment and estimate the person's prognosis.

- Staging systems for cancer have evolved over time and continue to change as scientists learn more about cancer.

- The TNM staging system is based on the size and/or extent (reach) of the primary tumor (T), whether cancer cells have spread to nearby (regional) lymph nodes (N), and whether metastasis (M), or the spread of the cancer to other parts of the body, has occurred.

- Physical exams, imaging procedures, laboratory tests, pathology reports, and surgical reports provide information to determine the stage of a cancer.

What is staging?

Staging describes the severity of a person's cancer based on the size and/or extent (reach) of the original (primary) tumor and whether or not cancer has spread in the body. Staging is important for several reasons:

- Staging helps the doctor plan the appropriate treatment.
- Cancer stage can be used in estimating a person's prognosis.
- Knowing the stage of cancer is important in identifying clinical trials that may be a suitable treatment option for a patient.
- Staging helps health care providers and researchers exchange information about patients; it also gives them a common terminology for evaluating the results of clinical trials and comparing the results of different trials.

Staging is based on knowledge of the way cancer progresses. Cancer cells grow and divide without control or order, and they do not die when they should. As a result, they often form a mass of tissue called a tumor. As a tumor grows, it can invade nearby tissues and organs. Cancer cells can also break away from a tumor and enter the bloodstream or the lymphatic system. By moving through the bloodstream or lymphatic system, cancer cells can spread from the primary site to lymph nodes or to other organs, where they may form new tumors. The spread of cancer is called metastasis.

What are the common elements of staging systems?

Staging systems for cancer have evolved over time. They continue to change as scientists learn more about cancer. Some staging systems cover many types of cancer; others focus on a particular type. The common elements considered in most staging systems are as follows:

- Site of the primary tumor and the cell type (e.g., adenocarcinoma, squamous cell carcinoma)
- Tumor size and/or extent (reach)
- Regional lymph node involvement (the spread of cancer to nearby lymph nodes)
- Number of tumors (the primary tumor and the presence of metastatic tumors, or metastases)
- Tumor grade* (how closely the cancer cells and tissue resemble normal cells and tissue)

What is the TNM system?

The TNM system is one of the most widely used cancer staging systems. This system has been accepted by the Union for International Cancer Control (UICC) and the American Joint Committee on Cancer (AJCC). Most medical facilities use the TNM system as their main method for cancer reporting.

The TNM system is based on the size and/or extent (reach) of the primary tumor (**T**), the amount of spread to nearby lymph nodes (**N**), and the presence of metastasis (**M**) or secondary tumors formed by the spread of cancer cells to other parts of the body. A number is added to each letter to indicate the size and/or extent of the primary tumor and the degree of cancer spread.

Primary Tumor (T)

TX: Primary tumor cannot be evaluated

T0: No evidence of primary tumor

Tis: Carcinoma in situ (CIS; abnormal cells are present but have not spread to neighboring tissue; although not cancer, CIS may become cancer and is sometimes called preinvasive cancer)

T1, T2, T3, T4: Size and/or extent of the primary tumor

Regional Lymph Nodes (N)

NX: Regional lymph nodes cannot be evaluated

N0: No regional lymph node involvement

N1, N2, N3: Degree of regional lymph node involvement (number and location of lymph nodes)

Distant Metastasis (M)

MX: Distant metastasis cannot be evaluated

M0: No distant metastasis

M1: Distant metastasis is present

For example, breast cancer classified as T3 N2 M0 refers to a large tumor that has spread outside the breast to nearby lymph nodes but not to other parts of the body. Prostate cancer T2 N0 M0 means that the tumor is located only in the prostate and has not spread to the lymph nodes or any other part of the body.

For many cancers, TNM combinations correspond to one of five stages. Criteria for stages differ for different types of cancer. For example, bladder cancer T3 N0 M0 is stage III, whereas colon cancer T3 N0 M0 is stage II.

Stage	Definition
Stage 0	Carcinoma in situ
Stage I, Stage II, and Stage III	Higher numbers indicate more extensive disease: Larger tumor size and/or spread of the cancer beyong the organ in which it first developed to nearby lymph nodes and/or tissues or organs adjacent to the location of the primary tumor
Stage IV	The cancer has spread to distant tissues or organs

Are all cancers staged with TNM classifications?

Most types of cancer have TNM designations, but some do not. For example, cancers of the brain and spinal cord are staged according to their cell type and grade. Different staging systems are also used for many cancers of the blood or bone marrow, such as lymphomas. The Ann Arbor staging classification is commonly used to stage lymphomas and has been adopted by both the AJCC and the UICC. However, other cancers of the blood or bone marrow, including most types of leukemia, do not have a clear-cut staging system. Another staging system, developed by the International Federation of Gynecology and Obstetrics (FIGO), is used to stage cancers of the cervix, uterus, ovary, vagina, and vulva. This system is also based on TNM information. Additionally, most childhood cancers are staged using either the TNM system or the staging criteria of the Children's Oncology Group (COG), which conducts pediatric clinical trials; however, other staging systems may be used for some childhood cancers.

Many cancer registries, such as those supported by NCI's Surveillance, Epidemiology, and End Results (SEER) Program, use "summary staging." This system is used for all types of cancer. It groups cancer cases into five main categories:

- *In situ*: Abnormal cells are present only in the layer of cells in which they developed
- *Localized*: Cancer is limited to the organ in which it began, without evidence of spread
- *Regional*: Cancer has spread beyond the primary site to nearby lymph nodes or tissues and organs
- *Distant*: Cancer has spread from the primary site to distant tissues or organs or to distant lymph nodes
- *Unknown*: There is not enough information to determine the stage

What types of tests are used to determine stage?

The types of tests used for staging depend on the type of cancer. Tests include the following:

- *Physical exams* are used to gather information about the cancer. The doctor examines the body by looking, feeling, and listening for anything unusual. The physical exam may show the location and size of the tumor(s) and the spread of the cancer to the lymph nodes and/or to other tissues and organs.
- *Imaging studies* produce pictures of areas inside the body. These studies are important tools in

determining stage. Procedures such as x-rays, computed tomography (CT) scans, magnetic resonance imaging (MRI) scans, and positron emission tomography (PET) scans can show the location of the cancer, the size of the tumor, and whether the cancer has spread.

- *Laboratory tests* are studies of blood, urine, other fluids, and tissues taken from the body. For example, tests for liver function and tumor markers (substances sometimes found in increased amounts if cancer is present) can provide information about the cancer.

- *Pathology reports* may include information about the size of the tumor, the growth of the tumor into other tissues and organs, the type of cancer cells, and the grade of the tumor. A biopsy may be performed to provide information for the pathology report. Cytology reports also describe findings from the examination of cells in body fluids.

- *Surgical reports* tell what is found during surgery. These reports describe the size and appearance of the tumor and often include observations about lymph nodes and nearby organs.

Chapter 3: Computed Tomography (CT) Scans

What is computed tomography?

Computed tomography (CT) is a diagnostic procedure that uses special x-ray equipment to obtain cross-sectional pictures of the body. The CT computer displays these pictures as detailed images of organs, bones, and other tissues. This procedure is also called CT scanning, computerized tomography, or computerized axial tomography (CAT).

How is CT used in cancer?

Computed tomography is used in several ways:

- To detect or confirm the presence of a tumor;
- To provide information about the size and location of the tumor and whether it has spread;
- To guide a biopsy (the removal of cells or tissues for examination under a microscope);
- To help plan radiation therapy or surgery; and
- To determine whether the cancer is responding to treatment.

What can a person expect during the CT procedure?

During a CT scan, the person lies very still on a table. The table slowly passes through the center of a large x-ray machine. The person might hear whirring sounds during the procedure. People may be asked to hold their breath at times, to prevent blurring of the pictures.

Often, a contrast agent, or "dye," may be given by mouth, injected into a vein, given by enema, or given in all three ways before the CT scan is done. The contrast dye can highlight specific areas inside the body, resulting in a clearer picture.

Computed tomography scans do not cause any pain. However, lying in one position during the procedure may be slightly uncomfortable. The length of the procedure depends on the size of the area being x-rayed; CT scans take from 15 minutes to 1 hour to complete. For most people, the CT scan is performed on an outpatient basis at a hospital or a doctor's office, without an overnight hospital stay.

Are there risks associated with a CT scan?

Some people may be concerned about the amount of radiation they receive during a CT scan. It is true that the radiation exposure from a CT scan can be higher than from a regular x-ray. However, not having the procedure can be more risky than having it, especially if cancer is suspected. People considering CT must weigh the risks and benefits. In very rare cases, contrast agents can cause allergic reactions. Some people experience mild itching or hives (small bumps on the skin). Symptoms of a more serious allergic reaction include shortness of breath and swelling of the throat or other parts of the body. People should tell the technologist immediately if they experience any of these symptoms, so they can be treated promptly.

What is spiral CT?

A spiral (or helical) CT scan is a new kind of CT. During a spiral CT, the x-ray machine rotates continuously around the body, following a spiral path to make cross-sectional pictures of the body. Benefits of spiral CT include:

- It can be used to make 3–dimensional pictures of areas inside the body;
- It may detect small abnormal areas better than conventional CT; and
- It is faster, so the test takes less time than a conventional CT.

What is total or whole body CT? Should a person have one?

A total or whole body CT scan creates images of nearly the entire body—from the chin to below the hips. This test has not been shown to have any value as a screening tool. ("Screening" means checking for signs of a disease when a person has no symptoms.)

The American College of Radiology (as well as most doctors) does not recommend scanning a person's body on the chance of finding signs of any sort of disease. In most cases abnormal findings do not indicate a serious health problem; however, a person must often undergo more tests to find this out. The additional tests can be expensive, inconvenient, and uncomfortable. The disadvantages of total body CT almost always outweigh the benefits.

What is virtual endoscopy?

Virtual endoscopy is a new technique that uses spiral CT. It allows doctors to see inside organs and other structures without surgery or special instruments. One type of virtual endoscopy, known as CT colonography or virtual colonoscopy, is under study as a screening technique for colon cancer.

What is combined PET/CT scanning?

Combined PET/CT scanning joins two imaging tests, CT and positron emission tomography (PET), into one procedure. A PET scan creates colored pictures of chemical changes (metabolic activity) in tissues. Because cancerous tumors usually are more active than normal tissue, they appear different on a PET scan.

Combining CT with PET scanning may provide a more complete picture of a tumor's location and growth or spread than either test alone. Researchers hope that the combined procedure will improve health care professionals' ability to diagnose cancer, determine how far it has spread, and follow patients' responses to treatment. The combined PET/CT scan may also reduce the number of additional imaging tests and other procedures a patient needs. However, this new technology is currently available only at some facilities.

Chapter 4: Mammograms

- A mammogram is an x-ray picture of the breast. Screening mammograms are used to check for breast cancer in women who have no signs or symptoms of the disease. Diagnostic mammograms are used to check for breast cancer after a lump or other sign or symptom of the disease has been found.

- Screening mammography can help reduce the number of deaths from breast cancer among women ages 40 to 70.

- Potential harms of screening mammography include false-negative results, false-positive results, overdiagnosis, overtreatment, and radiation exposure.

- NCI recommends that women age 40 or older have screening mammograms every 1 to 2 years.

What is a mammogram?

A mammogram is an x-ray picture of the breast. Mammograms can be used to check for breast cancer in women who have no signs or symptoms of the disease. This type of mammogram is called a screening mammogram.

Screening mammograms usually involve two x-ray pictures, or images, of each breast. The x-ray images make it possible to detect tumors that cannot be felt. Screening mammograms can also find microcalcifications (tiny deposits of calcium) that sometimes indicate the presence of breast cancer. Mammograms can also be used to check for breast cancer after a lump or other sign or symptom of the disease has been found. This type of mammogram is called a diagnostic mammogram. Besides a lump, signs of breast cancer can include breast pain, thickening of the skin of the breast, nipple discharge, or a change in breast size or shape; however, these signs may also be signs of benign conditions. A diagnostic mammogram can also be used to evaluate changes found during a screening mammogram or to view breast tissue when it is difficult to obtain a screening mammogram because of special circumstances, such as the presence of breast implants

How are screening and diagnostic mammograms different?

Diagnostic mammography takes longer than screening mammography because more x-rays are needed to obtain views of the breast from several angles. The technician may magnify a suspicious area to produce a detailed picture that can help the doctor make an accurate diagnosis.

What are the benefits of screening mammograms?

Early detection of breast cancer with screening mammography means that treatment can be started earlier in the course of the disease, possibly before it has spread. Results from randomized clinical trials and other studies show that screening mammography can help reduce the number of deaths from breast cancer among women ages 40 to 70, especially for those over age 50. However, studies to date have not shown a benefit from regular screening mammography in women under age 40 or from baseline screening mammograms (mammograms used for comparison) taken before age 40.

What are some of the potential harms of screening mammograms?

Finding cancer early does not always reduce a woman's chance of dying from breast cancer. Even though mammograms can detect malignant tumors that cannot be felt, treating a small tumor does not always mean that the woman will not die from the cancer. A fast-growing or aggressive cancer may have already spread to other parts of the body before it is detected. Women with such tumors live a longer period of time knowing that they likely have a fatal disease.

In addition, screening mammograms may not help prolong the life of a woman who is suffering from other, more life-threatening health conditions.

False-negative results

False-negative results occur when mammograms appear normal even though breast cancer is present. Overall, screening mammograms miss about 20 percent of breast cancers that are present at the time of screening.

The main cause of false-negative results is high breast density. Breasts contain both dense tissue (i.e., glandular tissue and connective tissue, together known as fibroglandular tissue) and fatty tissue. Fatty tissue appears dark on a mammogram, whereas fibroglandular tissue appears as white areas. Because fibroglandular tissue and tumors have similar density, tumors can be harder to detect in women with denser breasts.

False-negative results occur more often among younger women than among older women because younger women are more likely to have dense breasts. As a woman ages, her breasts usually become more fatty, and false-negative results become less likely. False-negative results can lead to delays in treatment and a false sense of security for affected women.

False-positive results

False-positive results occur when radiologists decide mammograms are abnormal but no cancer is actually present. All abnormal mammograms should be followed up with additional testing (diagnostic mammograms, ultrasound, and/or biopsy) to determine whether cancer is present.

False-positive results are more common for younger women, women who have had previous breast biopsies, women with a family history of breast cancer, and women who are taking estrogen (for example, menopausal hormone therapy).

False-positive mammogram results can lead to anxiety and other forms of psychological distress in affected women. The additional testing required to rule out cancer can also be costly and time consuming and can cause physical discomfort.

Overdiagnosis and overtreatment

Screening mammograms can find cancers and cases of ductal carcinoma in situ (DCIS, a noninvasive tumor in which abnormal cells that may become cancerous build up in the lining of breast ducts) that need to be treated. However, they can also find cancers and cases of DCIS that will never cause symptoms or threaten a woman's life, leading to "overdiagnosis" of breast cancer. Treatment of these latter cancers and cases of DCIS is not needed and leads to "overtreatment." Overtreatment exposes women unnecessarily to the adverse effects associated with cancer therapy.

Because doctors often cannot distinguish cancers and cases of DCIS that need to be treated from those that do not, they are all treated.

Radiation exposure

Mammograms require very small doses of radiation. The risk of harm from this radiation exposure is extremely low, but repeated x-rays have the potential to cause cancer. The benefits of mammography, however, nearly always outweigh the potential harm from the radiation exposure. Nevertheless, women should talk with their health care providers about the need for each x-ray. In addition, they should always let their health care provider and the x-ray technician know if there is any possibility that they are pregnant, because radiation can harm a growing fetus.

What are the National Cancer Institue's recommendations for screening mammograms?

- Women age 40 and older should have mammograms every 1 to 2 years.

- Women who are at higher than average risk of breast cancer (for example, because of a family history of the disease or because they carry a known mutation in either the BRCA1 or the BRCA2 gene) should talk with their health care providers about whether to have mammograms before age 40 and how often to have them.

What is the best method of detecting breast cancer as early as possible?

Getting a high-quality screening mammogram and having a clinical breast exam (an exam done by a health care provider) on a regular basis are the most effective ways to detect breast cancer early. As with any screening test, screening mammograms have both benefits and limitations. For example, some cancers cannot be detected by a screening mammogram but may be found by a clinical breast exam. Checking one's own breasts for lumps or other unusual changes is called a breast self-exam, or BSE. This type of exam cannot replace regular screening mammograms or clinical breast exams. In clinical trials, BSE alone was not found to help reduce the number of deaths from breast cancer.

Although regular BSE is not specifically recommended for breast cancer screening, many women choose to examine their own breasts. Women who do so should remember that breast changes can occur because of pregnancy, aging, menopause, during menstrual cycles, or when taking birth control pills or other hormones. It is normal for breasts to feel a little lumpy and uneven. Also, it is common for breasts to be swollen and tender right before or during a menstrual period. If a woman notices any unusual changes in her breasts, she should contact her health care provider.

What is the Breast Imaging Reporting and Database System (BI-RADS®)?

The American College of Radiology (ACR) has established a uniform way for radiologists to describe mammogram findings. The system, called BI-RADS, includes seven standardized categories, or levels. Each BI-RADS category has a follow-up plan associated with it to help radiologists and other physicians appropriately manage a patient's care.

Breast Imaging Reporting and Database System (BI-RADS)

Category	Assessment	Follow-up
0	Need additional imaging	Additional imaging needed before a category

	evaluation	can be assigned
1	Negative	Continue regular screening mammograms (for women over age 40)
2	Benign (noncancerous) finding	Continue regular screening mammograms (for women over age 40)
3	Probably benign	Receive a 6-month follow-up mammogram
4	Suspicious abnormality	May require biopsy
5	Highly suggestive of malignancy (cancer)	Requires biopsy
6	Known biopsy-proven malignancy (cancer)	Biopsy confirms presence of cancer before treatment begins

How much does a mammogram cost?

For most women with private insurance, the cost of screening mammograms is covered without copayments or deductibles, but women should contact their mammography facility or health insurance company for confirmation of the cost and coverage.

Medicare pays for annual screening mammograms for all female Medicare beneficiaries who are age 40 or older. Medicare will also pay for one baseline mammogram for female beneficiaries between the ages of 35 and 39. There is no deductible requirement for this benefit. Information about coverage is available through the Medicare Hotline at 1-800-MEDICARE (633-4227).

How can uninsured or low-income women obtain a free or low-cost screening mammogram?

Some state and local health programs and employers provide mammograms free or at low cost. For example, the Centers for Disease Control and Prevention (CDC) coordinates the National Breast and Cervical Cancer Early Detection Program. This program provides screening services, including clinical breast exams and mammograms, to low-income, uninsured women throughout the United States and in several U.S. territories. Contact information for local programs is available by calling 1-800-CDC-INFO (232-4636).

Information about free or low-cost mammography screening programs is also available from The National Cancer

Institute's Cancer Information Service at 1–800–4–CANCER (422–6237) and from local hospitals, health departments, women's centers, or other community groups.

Where can women get high-quality mammograms?

Women can get high-quality mammograms in breast clinics, hospital radiology departments, mobile vans, private radiology offices, and doctors' offices.

The Mammography Quality Standards Act (MQSA) is a Federal law that requires mammography facilities across the nation to meet uniform quality standards. Under the law, all mammography facilities must: 1) be accredited by an FDA-approved accreditation body; 2) be certified by the FDA, or an agency of a state that has been approved by the FDA, as meeting the standards; 3) undergo an annual MQSA inspection; and 4) prominently display the certificate issued by the agency.

Women can ask their doctors or staff at a local mammography facility about FDA certification before making an appointment. Women should look for the MQSA certificate at the mammography facility and check its expiration date. MQSA regulations also require that mammography facilities give patients an easy-to-read report of their mammogram results.

What should women with breast implants do about screening mammograms?

Women with breast implants should continue to have mammograms. (A woman who had an implant following a mastectomy should ask her doctor whether a mammogram of the reconstructed breast is necessary.) It is important to let the mammography facility know about breast implants when scheduling a mammogram. The technician and radiologist must be experienced in performing mammography on women who have breast implants. Implants can hide some breast tissue, making it more difficult for the radiologist to detect an abnormality on the mammogram. If the technician performing the procedure is aware that a woman has breast implants, steps can be taken to make sure that as much breast tissue as possible can be seen on the mammogram. A special technique called implant displacement views may be used.

What is digital mammography? How is it different from conventional (film) mammography?

Digital and conventional mammography both use x-rays to produce an image of the breast; however, in conventional mammography, the image is stored directly on film, whereas, in digital mammography, an electronic image of the breast is stored as a computer file. This digital information can be enhanced, magnified, or manipulated for further evaluation more easily than information stored on film.

Because digital mammography allows a radiologist to adjust, store, and retrieve digital images electronically, digital mammography may offer the following advantages over conventional mammography:

- Health care providers can share image files electronically, making long-distance consultations between radiologists and breast surgeons easier.
- Subtle differences between normal and abnormal tissues may be more easily noted.
- Fewer follow-up procedures may be needed.
- Fewer repeat images may be needed, reducing the exposure to radiation.

To date there is no evidence that digital mammography helps to further reduce a woman's risk of dying from breast cancer. Results from a large NCI-sponsored clinical trial that compared digital mammography with film mammography found no difference between digital and film mammograms in detecting breast cancer in the general population of women in the trial; however, digital mammography appeared to be more accurate than conventional film mammography in younger women with dense breasts. A subsequent analysis of women aged 40 through 79 who were undergoing screening in U.S. community-based imaging facilities also found that digital and film mammography had similar accuracy in most women. Digital screening had higher sensitivity in women with dense breasts.

Some health care providers recommend that women who have a very high risk of breast cancer, such as those with a known mutation in either the BRCA1 or BRCA2 gene or extremely dense breasts, have digital mammograms instead of conventional mammograms; however, no studies have shown that digital mammograms are superior to conventional mammograms in reducing the risk of death for these women. Digital mammography can be done only in facilities that are certified to practice conventional mammography and have received FDA approval to offer digital mammography. The procedure for having a mammogram with a digital system is the same as with conventional mammography.

What is 3D mammography?

Three-dimensional (3D) mammography, also known as breast tomosynthesis, is a type of digital mammography in which x-ray machines are used to take pictures of thin slices of the breast from different angles and computer software is used to reconstruct an image. This process is similar to how a computed tomography (CT) scanner produces images of structures inside of the body. 3D mammography uses very low dose x-rays, but, because it is generally performed at the same time as standard two-dimensional (2D) digital mammography, the radiation dose is slightly higher than that of standard mammography. The accuracy of 3D mammography has not been compared with that of 2D mammography in randomized studies. Therefore, researchers do not know whether 3D mammography is better or worse than standard mammography at avoiding false-positive results and identifying early cancers.

What other technologies are being developed for breast cancer screening?

The National Cancer Institute is supporting the development of several new technologies to detect breast tumors. This research ranges from methods being developed in research labs to those that are being studied in clinical trials. Efforts to improve conventional mammography include digital mammography, magnetic resonance imaging (MRI), positron emission tomography (PET) scanning, and diffuse optical tomography, which uses light instead of x-rays to create pictures of the breast.

Chapter 5: Interpreting Laboratory Test Results

A laboratory test is a medical procedure in which a sample of blood, urine, or other tissues or substances in the body is checked for certain features. Such tests are often used as part of a routine checkup to identify possible changes in a person's health before any symptoms appear. Laboratory tests also play an important role in diagnosis when a person has symptoms. In addition, tests may be used to help plan a patient's treatment, evaluate the response to treatment, or monitor the course of the disease over time.

Laboratory test samples are analyzed to determine whether the results fall within normal ranges. They also may be checked for changes from previous tests. Normal test values are usually given as a range, rather than as a specific number, because normal values vary from person to person. What is normal for one person may not be normal for another person. Many factors (including the patient's sex, age, race, medical history, and general health) can affect test results.

Sometimes, test results are affected by specific foods, drugs the patient is taking, and how closely the patient follows pre-test instructions. That is why a patient may be asked not to eat or drink for several hours before a test. It is also common for normal ranges to vary somewhat from laboratory to laboratory.

Some laboratory tests are precise, reliable indicators of specific health problems. Others provide more general information that simply gives doctors clues to possible health problems. Information obtained from laboratory tests may help doctors decide whether other tests or procedures are needed to make a diagnosis. The information may also help the doctor develop or revise a patient's treatment plan. All laboratory test results must be interpreted in the context of the overall health of the patient and are generally used along with other exams or tests. The doctor who is familiar with the patient's medical history and current condition is in the best position to explain test results and their implications. Patients are encouraged to discuss questions or concerns about laboratory test results with the doctor.

Chapter 6: Pathology Reports

- A pathology report is a document that contains the diagnosis determined by examining cells and tissues under a microscope.

- Frozen sections of a tissue sample are done when an immediate answer about a sample is needed.

- The pathology report is usually created after a biopsy or surgery.

- The pathology report includes information about the patient, a description of how cells look under the microscope, and a diagnosis.

- The National Cancer Institute is sponsoring clinical trials that are designed to improve the accuracy and specificity of cancer diagnoses.

What is a pathology report?

A pathology report is a document that contains the diagnosis determined by examining cells and tissues under a microscope. The report may also contain information about the size, shape, and appearance of a specimen as it looks to the naked eye. This information is known as the gross description.

A pathologist is a doctor who does this examination and writes the pathology report. Pathology reports play an important role in cancer diagnosis and staging (describing the extent of cancer within the body, especially whether it has spread), which helps determine treatment options.

How is tissue obtained for examination by the pathologist?

In most cases, a doctor needs to do a biopsy or surgery to remove cells or tissues for examination under a microscope. Some common ways a biopsy can be done are as follows:

- A needle is used to withdraw tissue or fluid.
- An endoscope (a thin, lighted tube) is used to look at areas inside the body and remove cells or tissues.
- Surgery is used to remove part of the tumor or the entire tumor. If the entire tumor is removed, typically some normal tissue around the tumor is also removed.

Tissue removed during a biopsy is sent to a pathology laboratory, where it is sliced into thin sections for viewing under a microscope. This is known as histologic (tissue) examination and is usually the best way to tell if cancer is present. The pathologist may also examine cytologic (cell) material. Cytologic material is present in urine, cerebrospinal fluid (the fluid around the brain and spinal cord), sputum (mucus from the lungs), peritoneal (abdominal cavity) fluid, pleural (chest cavity) fluid, cervical/vaginal smears, and in fluid removed during a biopsy.

How is tissue processed after a biopsy or surgery? What is a frozen section?

The tissue removed during a biopsy or surgery must be cut into thin sections, placed on slides, and stained with dyes before it can be examined under a microscope. Two methods are used to make the tissue firm enough to cut into thin sections: frozen sections and paraffin-embedded (permanent) sections. All tissue samples are prepared as permanent sections, but sometimes frozen sections are also prepared. Permanent sections are prepared by placing the tissue in fixative (usually formalin) to preserve the tissue, processing it through additional solutions, and then placing it in paraffin wax. After the wax has hardened, the tissue is cut into very thin slices, which are placed on slides and stained. The process normally takes several days. A permanent section provides the best quality for examination by the pathologist and produces more accurate results than a frozen section.

Frozen sections are prepared by freezing and slicing the tissue sample. They can be done in about 15 to 20 minutes while the patient is in the operating room. Frozen sections are done when an immediate answer is needed; for example, to determine whether the tissue is cancerous so as to guide the surgeon during the course of an operation.

How long after the tissue sample is taken will the pathology report be ready?

The pathologist sends a pathology report to the doctor within 10 days after the biopsy or surgery is performed. Pathology reports are written in technical medical language. Patients may want to ask their doctors to give them a copy of the pathology report and to explain the report to them. Patients also may wish to keep a copy of their pathology report in their own records.

What information does a pathology report usually include?

The pathology report may include the following information:

- *Patient information*: Name, birth date, biopsy date
- *Gross description*: Color, weight, and size of tissue as seen by the naked eye

- *Microscopic description*: How the sample looks under the microscope and how it compares with normal cells
- *Diagnosis*: Type of tumor/cancer and grade (how abnormal the cells look under the microscope and how quickly the tumor is likely to grow and spread)
- *Tumor size*: Measured in centimeters
- *Tumor margins*: There are three possible findings when the biopsy sample is the entire tumor:
  - *Positive margins* mean that cancer cells are found at the edge of the material removed
  - *Negative, not involved, clear, or free margins* mean that no cancer cells are found at the outer edge
  - *Close margins* are neither negative nor positive
- *Other information*: Usually notes about samples that have been sent for other tests or a second opinion
- Pathologist's signature and name and address of the laboratory

What might the pathology report say about the physical and chemical characteristics of the tissue?

After identifying the tissue as cancerous, the pathologist may perform additional tests to get more information about the tumor that cannot be determined by looking at the tissue with routine stains, such as hematoxylin and eosin (also known as H&E), under a microscope. The pathology report will include the results of these tests. For example, the pathology report may include information obtained from immunochemical stains (IHC). IHC uses antibodies to identify specific antigens on the surface of cancer cells. IHC can often be used to:

- Determine where the cancer started
- Distinguish among different cancer types, such as carcinoma, melanoma, and lymphoma
- Help diagnose and classify leukemias and lymphomas

The pathology report may also include the results of flow cytometry. Flow cytometry is a method of measuring properties of cells in a sample, including the number of cells, percentage of live cells, cell size and shape, and presence of tumor markers on the cell surface. Tumor markers are substances produced by tumor cells or by other cells in the body in response to cancer or certain noncancerous conditions.) Flow cytometry can be used in the diagnosis, classification, and management of cancers such as acute leukemia, chronic lymphoproliferative disorders, and non-Hodgkin lymphoma.

Finally, the pathology report may include the results of molecular diagnostic and cytogenetic studies. Such studies investigate the presence or absence of malignant cells, and genetic or molecular abnormalities in specimens.

What information about the genetics of the cells might be included in the pathology report?

Cytogenetics uses tissue culture and specialized techniques to provide genetic information about cells, particularly genetic alterations. Some genetic alterations are markers or indicators of a specific cancer. For example, the Philadelphia chromosome is associated with chronic myelogenous leukemia (CML). Some alterations can provide information about prognosis, which helps the doctor make treatment recommendations. Some tests that might be performed on a tissue sample include:

- *Fluorescence in situ hybridization (FISH)*: Determines the positions of particular genes. It can be used to identify chromosomal abnormalities and to map genes.

- *Polymerase chain reaction (PCR):* A method of making many copies of particular DNA sequences of relevance to the diagnosis.
- *Real-time PCR or quantitative PCR*: A method of measuring how many copies of a particular DNA sequence are present.
- *Reverse-transcriptase polymerase chain reaction (RT-PCR):* A method of making many copies of a specific RNA sequence.
- *Southern blot hybridization*: Detects specific DNA fragments.
- *Western blot hybridization*: Identifies and analyzes proteins or peptides.

Can individuals get a second opinion about their pathology results?

Although most cancers can be easily diagnosed, sometimes patients or their doctors may want to get a second opinion about the pathology results. Patients interested in getting a second opinion should talk with their doctor. They will need to obtain the slides and/or paraffin block from the pathologist who examined the sample or from the hospital where the biopsy or surgery was done.

Many institutions provide second opinions on pathology specimens.

Chapter 7: Tumor Markers

- Tumor markers are substances found in the blood, urine, stool, other bodily fluids, or tissues of some patients with cancer.
- Tumor markers may be used to help diagnose cancer, predict a patient's response to certain cancer therapies, check a patient's response to treatment, or determine whether cancer has returned.
- More than 20 tumor markers are currently in use.

What are tumor markers?

Tumor markers are substances that are produced by cancer or by other cells of the body in response to cancer or certain benign (noncancerous) conditions. Most tumor markers are made by normal cells as well as by cancer cells; however, they are produced at much higher levels in cancerous conditions. These substances can be found in the blood, urine, stool, tumor tissue, or other tissues or bodily fluids of some patients with cancer. Most tumor markers are proteins. However, more recently, patterns of gene expression and changes to DNA have also begun to be used as tumor markers. Markers of the latter type are assessed in tumor tissue specifically.

Thus far, more than 20 different tumor markers have been characterized and are in clinical use. Some are associated with only one type of cancer, whereas others are associated with two or more cancer types. There is no "universal" tumor marker that can detect any type of cancer.

There are some limitations to the use of tumor markers. Sometimes, noncancerous conditions can cause the levels of certain tumor markers to increase. In addition, not everyone with a particular type of cancer will have a higher level of a tumor marker associated with that cancer. Moreover, tumor markers have not been identified for every type of cancer.

How are tumor markers used in cancer care?

Tumor markers are used to help detect, diagnose, and manage some types of cancer. Although an elevated level of a tumor marker may suggest the presence of cancer, this alone is not enough to diagnose cancer. Therefore, measurements of tumor markers are usually combined with other tests, such as biopsies, to diagnose cancer.

Tumor marker levels may be measured before treatment to help doctors plan the appropriate therapy. In some types of cancer, the level of a tumor marker reflects the stage (extent) of the disease and/or the patient's prognosis (likely outcome or course of disease).

Tumor markers may also be measured periodically during cancer therapy. A decrease in the level of a tumor marker or a return to the marker's normal level may indicate that the cancer is responding to treatment, whereas no change or an increase may indicate that the cancer is not responding. Tumor markers may also be measured after treatment has ended to check for recurrence (the return of cancer).

How are tumor markers measured?

A doctor takes a sample of tumor tissue or bodily fluid and sends it to a laboratory, where various methods are used to measure the level of the tumor marker.

If the tumor marker is being used to determine whether treatment is working or whether there is a recurrence, the marker's level will be measured in multiple samples taken over time. Usually these "serial measurements," which show whether the level of a marker is increasing, staying the same, or decreasing, are more meaningful than a single measurement.

What tumor markers are currently being used, and for which cancer types?

A number of tumor markers are currently being used for a wide range of cancer types. Although most of these can be tested in laboratories that meet standards set by the Clinical Laboratory Improvement Amendments, some cannot be and may therefore be considered experimental. Tumor markers that are currently in common use are listed below.

ALK gene rearrangements

- Cancer types: Non-small cell lung cancer and anaplastic large cell lymphoma
- Tissue analyzed: Tumor
- How used: To help determine treatment and prognosis

Alpha-fetoprotein (AFP)

- Cancer types: Liver cancer and germ cell tumors
- Tissue analyzed: Blood
- How used: To help diagnose liver cancer and follow response to treatment; to assess stage, prognosis, and response to treatment of germ cell tumors

Beta-2-microglobulin (B2M)

- Cancer types: Multiple myeloma, chronic lymphocytic leukemia, and some lymphomas
- Tissue analyzed: Blood, urine, or cerebrospinal fluid

- How used: To determine prognosis and follow response to treatment

Beta-human chorionic gonadotropin (Beta-hCG)

- Cancer types: Choriocarcinoma and testicular cancer
- Tissue analyzed: Urine or blood
- How used: To assess stage, prognosis, and response to treatment

BCR-ABL fusion gene

- Cancer type: Chronic myeloid leukemia
- Tissue analyzed: Blood and/or bone marrow
- How used: To confirm diagnosis and monitor disease status

BRAF mutation V600E

- Cancer types: Cutaneous melanoma and colorectal cancer
- Tissue analyzed: Tumor
- How used: To predict response to targeted therapies

CA15-3/CA27.29

- Cancer type: Breast cancer
- Tissue analyzed: Blood
- How used: To assess whether treatment is working or disease has recurred

CA19-9

- Cancer types: Pancreatic cancer, gallbladder cancer, bile duct cancer, and gastric cancer
- Tissue analyzed: Blood
- How used: To assess whether treatment is working

CA-125

- Cancer type: Ovarian cancer
- Tissue analyzed: Blood
- How used: To help in diagnosis, assessment of response to treatment, and evaluation of recurrence

Calcitonin

- Cancer type: Medullary thyroid cancer
- Tissue analyzed: Blood
- How used: To aid in diagnosis, check whether treatment is working, and assess recurrence

Carcinoembryonic antigen (CEA)

- Cancer types: Colorectal cancer and breast cancer
- Tissue analyzed: Blood
- How used: To check whether colorectal cancer has spread; to look for breast cancer recurrence and assess response to treatment

CD20

- Cancer type: Non-Hodgkin lymphoma
- Tissue analyzed: Blood
- How used: To determine whether treatment with a targeted therapy is appropriate

Chromogranin A (CgA)

- Cancer type: Neuroendocrine tumors
- Tissue analyzed: Blood
- How used: To help in diagnosis, assessment of treatment response, and evaluation of recurrence

Chromosomes 3, 7, 17, and 9p21

- Cancer type: Bladder cancer
- Tissue analyzed: Urine
- How used: To help in monitoring for tumor recurrence

Cytokeratin fragments 21-1

- Cancer type: Lung cancer
- Tissue analyzed: Blood
- How used: To help in monitoring for recurrence

EGFR mutation analysis

- Cancer type: Non-small cell lung cancer
- Tissue analyzed: Tumor
- How used: To help determine treatment and prognosis

Estrogen receptor (ER)/progesterone receptor (PR)

- Cancer type: Breast cancer
- Tissue analyzed: Tumor
- How used: To determine whether treatment with hormonal therapy (such as tamoxifen) is appropriate

Fibrin/fibrinogen

- Cancer type: Bladder cancer
- Tissue analyzed: Urine
- How used: To monitor progression and response to treatment

HE4

- Cancer type: Ovarian cancer
- Tissue analyzed: Blood
- How used: To assess disease progression and monitor for recurrence

HER2/neu

- Cancer types: Breast cancer, gastric cancer, and esophageal cancer
- Tissue analyzed: Tumor
- How used: To determine whether treatment with trastuzumab is appropriate

Immunoglobulins

- Cancer types: Multiple myeloma and Waldenström macroglobulinemia

- Tissue analyzed: Blood and urine
- How used: To help diagnose disease, assess response to treatment, and look for recurrence

KIT

- Cancer types: Gastrointestinal stromal tumor and mucosal melanoma
- Tissue analyzed: Tumor
- How used: To help in diagnosing and determining treatment

KRAS mutation analysis

- Cancer types: Colorectal cancer and non-small cell lung cancer
- Tissue analyzed: Tumor
- How used: To determine whether treatment with a particular type of targeted therapy is appropriate

Lactate dehydrogenase

- Cancer type: Germ cell tumors
- Tissue analyzed: Blood
- How used: To assess stage, prognosis, and response to treatment

Nuclear matrix protein 22

- Cancer type: Bladder cancer
- Tissue analyzed: Urine
- How used: To monitor response to treatment

Prostate-specific antigen (PSA)

- Cancer type: Prostate cancer
- Tissue analyzed: Blood
- How used: To help in diagnosis, assess response to treatment, and look for recurrence

Thyroglobulin

- Cancer type: Thyroid cancer
- Tissue analyzed: Tumor
- How used: To evaluate response to treatment and look for recurrence

Urokinase plasminogen activator (uPA) and plasminogen activator inhibitor (PAI-1)

- Cancer type: Breast cancer
- Tissue analyzed: Tumor
- How used: To determine aggressiveness of cancer and guide treatment

5-Protein signature (Ova1)

- Cancer type: Ovarian cancer
- Tissue analyzed: Blood
- How used: To pre-operatively assess pelvic mass for suspected ovarian cancer

21-Gene signature (Oncotype DX)

- Cancer type: Breast cancer
- Tissue analyzed: Tumor

- How used: To evaluate risk of recurrence

70-Gene signature (Mammaprint)

- Cancer type: Breast cancer
- Tissue analyzed: Tumor
- How used: To evaluate risk of recurrence

Can tumor markers be used in cancer screening?

Because tumor markers can be used to assess the response of a tumor to treatment and for prognosis, researchers have hoped that they might also be useful in screening tests that aim to detect cancer early, before there are any symptoms. For a screening test to be useful, it should have very high sensitivity (ability to correctly identify people who have the disease) and specificity (ability to correctly identify people who do not have the disease). If a test is highly sensitive, it will identify most people with the disease—that is, it will result in very few false-negative results. If a test is highly specific, only a small number of people will test positive for the disease who do not have it—in other words, it will result in very few false-positive results.

Although tumor markers are extremely useful in determining whether a tumor is responding to treatment or assessing whether it has recurred, no tumor marker identified to date is sufficiently sensitive or specific to be used on its own to screen for cancer.

For example, the prostate-specific antigen (PSA) test, which measures the level of PSA in the blood, is often used to screen men for prostate cancer. However, an increased PSA level can be caused by benign prostate conditions as well as by prostate cancer, and most men with an elevated PSA level do not have prostate cancer. Initial results from two large randomized controlled trials, the NCI-conducted Prostate, Lung, Colorectal, and Ovarian Cancer Screening Trial, or PLCO, and the European Randomized Study of Screening for Prostate Cancer, showed that PSA testing at best leads to only a small reduction in the number of prostate cancer deaths. Moreover, it is not clear whether the benefits of PSA screening outweigh the harms of follow-up diagnostic tests and treatments for cancers that in many cases would never have threatened a man's life.

Similarly, results from the PLCO trial showed that CA-125, a tumor marker that is sometimes elevated in the blood of women with ovarian cancer but can also be elevated in women with benign conditions, is not sufficiently sensitive or specific to be used together with transvaginal ultrasound to screen for ovarian cancer in women at average risk of the disease. An analysis of 28 potential markers for ovarian cancer in blood from women who later went on to develop ovarian cancer found that none of these markers performed even as well as CA-125 at detecting the disease in women at average risk.

What kind of research is under way to develop more accurate tumor markers?

Cancer researchers are turning to proteomics (the study of protein structure, function, and patterns of expression) in hopes of developing new biomarkers that can be used to identify disease in its early stages, to predict the effectiveness of treatment, or to predict the chance of cancer recurrence after treatment has ended.

Scientists are also evaluating patterns of gene expression for their ability to help determine a patient's prognosis or response to therapy. For example, the National Cancer Institute-sponsored TAILORx trial assigned women with lymph node-negative, hormone receptor–positive breast cancer who have undergone surgery to different treatments based on their recurrence scores in the Oncotype DX test. One of the goals of the trial is to determine whether women whose score indicates that they have an intermediate risk of recurrence will benefit from the addition of chemotherapy to hormonal therapy or whether such women can safely avoid chemotherapy. The trial has accrued its required number of subjects and these subjects will be followed for several years before results are available.

The Program for the Assessment of Clinical Cancer Tests (PACCT), an initiative of the Cancer Diagnosis Program of NCI's Division of Cancer Diagnosis and Treatment, has been developed to ensure that development of the next generation of laboratory tests is efficient and effective. The PACCT strategy group, which includes scientists from academia, industry, and NCI, is developing criteria for assessing which markers are ready for further development. PACCT also aims to improve access to human specimens, make standardized reagents and control materials, and support validation studies. A new program, the Clinical Assay Development Program, allows NCI to assist in the development of promising assays that may predict which treatment may be better or that will help indicate a particular cancer's aggressiveness.

Chapter 8: Tumor Grade

- Tumor grade is the description of a tumor based on how abnormal the tumor cells and tumor tissue look under a microscope.
- Tumor grade is an indicator of how quickly the tumor is likely to grow and spread.
- Tumor grading systems differ depending on the type of cancer.
- Tumor grade may be one of the factors considered when planning treatment for a patient.

What is tumor grade?

Tumor grade is the description of a tumor based on how abnormal the tumor cells and the tumor tissue look under a microscope. It is an indicator of how quickly a tumor is likely to grow and spread. If the cells of the tumor and the organization of the tumor's tissue are close to those of normal cells and tissue, the tumor is called "well-differentiated." These tumors tend to grow and spread at a slower rate than tumors that are "undifferentiated" or "poorly differentiated," which have abnormal-looking cells and may lack normal tissue structures. Based on these and other differences in microscopic appearance, doctors assign a numerical "grade" to most cancers. The factors used to determine tumor grade can vary between different types of cancer.

Tumor grade is not the same as the stage of a cancer. Cancer stage refers to the size and/or extent (reach) of the original (primary) tumor and whether or not cancer cells have spread in the body. Cancer stage is based on factors such as the location of the primary tumor, tumor size, regional lymph node involvement (the spread of cancer to nearby lymph nodes), and the number of tumors present.

How is tumor grade determined?

If a tumor is suspected to be malignant, a doctor removes all or part of it during a procedure called a biopsy. A pathologist (a doctor who identifies diseases by studying cells and tissues under a microscope) then examines the biopsied tissue to determine whether the tumor is benign or malignant. The pathologist also determines the tumor's grade and identifies other characteristics of the tumor.

How are tumor grades classified?

Grading systems differ depending on the type of cancer. In general, tumors are graded as 1, 2, 3, or 4, depending on the amount of abnormality. In Grade 1 tumors, the tumor cells and the organization of the tumor tissue appear close to normal. These tumors tend to grow and spread slowly. In contrast, the cells and tissue of Grade 3 and Grade 4 tumors do not look like normal cells and tissue. Grade 3 and Grade 4 tumors tend to grow rapidly and spread faster than tumors with a lower grade.

If a grading system for a tumor type is not specified, the following system is generally used (1):

- *GX*: Grade cannot be assessed (undetermined grade)
- *G1*: Well differentiated (low grade)
- *G2*: Moderately differentiated (intermediate grade)
- *G3*: Poorly differentiated (high grade)
- *G4*: Undifferentiated (high grade)

What are some of the cancer type-specific grading systems?

Breast and prostate cancers are the most common types of cancer that have their own grading systems.

Breast Cancer

Doctors most often use the Nottingham grading system (also called the Elston-Ellis modification of the Scarff-Bloom-

Richardson grading system) for breast cancer. This system grades breast tumors based on the following features:

- *Tubule formation*: how much of the tumor tissue has normal breast (milk) duct structures
- *Nuclear grade*: an evaluation of the size and shape of the nucleus in the tumor cells
- *Mitotic rate*: how many dividing cells are present, which is a measure of how fast the tumor cells are growing and dividing

Each of the categories gets a score between 1 and 3; a score of "1" means the cells and tumor tissue look the most like normal cells and tissue, and a score of "3" means the cells and tissue look the most abnormal. The scores for the three categories are then added, yielding a total score of 3 to 9. Three grades are possible:

- Total score = 3–5: G1 (Low grade or well differentiated)
- Total score = 6–7: G2 (Intermediate grade or moderately differentiated)
- Total score = 8–9: G3 (High grade or poorly differentiated)

Prostate Cancer

The Gleason scoring system is used to grade prostate cancer (1). The Gleason score is based on biopsy samples taken from the prostate. The pathologist checks the samples to see how similar the tumor tissue looks to normal prostate tissue. Both a primary and a secondary pattern of tissue organization are identified. The primary pattern represents the most common tissue pattern seen in the tumor, and the secondary pattern represents the next most common pattern. Each pattern is given a grade from 1 to 5, with 1 looking the most like normal prostate tissue and 5 looking the most abnormal. The two grades are then added to give a Gleason score. The American Joint Committee on Cancer recommends grouping Gleason scores into the following categories:

- *Gleason X*: Gleason score cannot be determined
- *Gleason 2–6*: The tumor tissue is well differentiated
- *Gleason 7*: The tumor tissue is moderately differentiated
- *Gleason 8–10*: The tumor tissue is poorly differentiated or undifferentiated

How does tumor grade affect a patient's treatment options?

Doctors use tumor grade and other factors, such as cancer stage and a patient's age and general health, to develop a treatment plan and to determine a patient's prognosis (the likely outcome or course of a disease; the chance of recovery or recurrence). Generally, a lower grade indicates a better prognosis. A higher-grade cancer may grow and spread more quickly and may require immediate or more aggressive treatment.

The importance of tumor grade in planning treatment and determining a patient's prognosis is greater for certain types of cancer, such as soft tissue sarcoma, primary brain tumors, and breast and prostate cancer.

Patients should talk with their doctor for more information about tumor grade and how it relates to their treatment and prognosis.

Chapter 9: Sentinel Lymph Node Biopsy

- A sentinel lymph node is the first lymph node(s) to which cancer cells are most likely to spread from a primary tumor.
- A sentinel lymph node biopsy (SLNB) can be used to help determine the extent, or stage, of cancer in the body.
- Because SLNBs involve less extensive surgery and the removal of fewer lymph nodes than standard lymph node surgery, the potential for adverse effects, or harms, is lower.

What are lymph nodes?

Lymph nodes are small round organs that are part of the body's lymphatic system. They are found widely throughout the body and are connected to one another by lymph vessels. Groups of lymph nodes are located in the neck, underarms, chest, abdomen, and groin. A clear fluid called lymph flows through lymph vessels and lymph nodes.

Lymph originates from a fluid, known as interstitial fluid, that has diffused, or "leaked," out of small blood vessels called capillaries. This fluid contains many substances, including blood plasma, proteins, glucose, and oxygen. It bathes most of the body's cells, providing them with the oxygen and nutrients they need for growth and survival. Interstitial fluid also picks up waste products from cells as well as other materials, such as bacteria and viruses, to help remove them from the body's tissues. Interstitial fluid eventually collects in lymph vessels, where it becomes known as lymph. Lymph flows through the body's lymph vessels to reach two large ducts at the base of the neck, where it is emptied into the bloodstream.

Lymph nodes are important parts of the body's immune system. They contain B lymphocytes, T lymphocytes, and other types of immune system cells. These cells monitor lymph for the presence of "foreign" substances, such as bacteria and viruses. If a foreign substance is detected, some of the cells will become activated and an immune response will be triggered.

Lymph nodes are also important in helping to determine whether cancer cells have developed the ability to spread to other parts of the body. Many types of cancer spread through the lymphatic system, and one of the earliest sites of spread for these cancers is nearby lymph nodes.

What is a sentinel lymph node?

A sentinel lymph node is defined as the first lymph node to which cancer cells are most likely to spread from a primary tumor. Sometimes, there can be more than one sentinel lymph node.

What is a sentinel lymph node biopsy?

A sentinel lymph node biopsy (SLNB) is a procedure in which the sentinel lymph node is identified, removed, and examined to determine whether cancer cells are present. A negative SLNB result suggests that cancer has not developed the ability to spread to nearby lymph nodes or other organs. A positive SLNB result indicates that cancer is present in the sentinel lymph node and may be present in other nearby lymph nodes (called regional lymph nodes) and, possibly, other organs. This information can help a doctor determine the stage of the cancer (extent of the disease within the body) and develop an appropriate treatment plan.

What happens during an SLNB?

A surgeon injects a radioactive substance, a blue dye, or both near the tumor to locate the position of the sentinel lymph node. The surgeon then uses a device that detects radioactivity to find the sentinel node or looks for lymph nodes that are stained with the blue dye. Once the sentinel lymph node is located, the surgeon makes a small incision (about 1/2 inch) in the overlying skin and removes the node. The sentinel node is then checked for the presence of cancer cells by a pathologist. If cancer is found, the surgeon may remove additional lymph nodes, either during the same biopsy procedure or during a follow-up surgical procedure. SLNBs may be done on an outpatient basis or may require a short stay in the hospital.

SLNB is usually done at the same time the primary tumor is removed. However, the procedure can also be done either before or after removal of the tumor.

What are the benefits of SLNB?

In addition to helping doctors stage cancers and estimate the risk that tumor cells have developed the ability to spread to other parts of the body, SLNB may help some patients avoid more extensive lymph node surgery. Removing additional nearby lymph nodes to look for cancer cells may not be necessary if the sentinel node is negative for cancer. All lymph node surgery can have adverse effects, and some of these effects may be reduced or avoided if fewer lymph nodes are removed. The potential adverse effects of lymph node surgery include the following:

- Lymphedema, or tissue swelling. During SLNB or more extensive lymph node surgery, lymph vessels leading to and from the sentinel node or group of nodes are cut, thereby disrupting the normal flow of lymph through the affected area. This disruption may lead to an abnormal buildup of lymph fluid. In addition to swelling, patients with lymphedema may experience pain or discomfort in the affected area, and the overlying skin may become thickened or hard. In the case of extensive lymph node surgery in an armpit or groin, the swelling may affect an entire arm or leg. In addition, there is an increased risk of infection in the affected area or limb. Very rarely, chronic lymphedema due to extensive lymph node removal may cause a cancer of the lymphatic vessels called lymphangiosarcoma.
- Seroma, or the buildup of lymph fluid at the site of the surgery.
- Numbness, tingling, or pain at the site of the surgery.
- Difficulty moving the affected body part.

Is SLNB associated with other harms?

SLNB, like other surgical procedures, can cause short-term pain, swelling, and bruising at the surgical site and increase the risk of infection. In addition, some patients may have skin or allergic reactions to the blue dye used in SLNB. Another potential harm is a false-negative biopsy result—that is, cancer cells are not seen in the sentinel lymph node although they are present and may have already spread to other regional lymph nodes or other parts of the body. A false-negative biopsy result gives the patient and the doctor a false sense of security about the extent of cancer in the patient's body.

Is SLNB used to help stage all types of cancer?

No. SLNB is most commonly used to help stage breast cancer and melanoma. However, it is being studied with other cancer types, including colorectal cancer, gastric cancer, esophageal cancer, head and neck cancer, thyroid cancer, and non-small cell lung cancer.

What has research shown about the use of SLNB in breast cancer?

Breast cancer cells are most likely to spread first to lymph nodes located in the axilla, or armpit area, next to the affected breast. However, in breast cancers close to the center of the chest (near the breastbone), cancer cells may spread first to lymph nodes inside the chest (under the breastbone) before they can be detected in the axilla.

The number of lymph nodes in the axilla varies from person to person but usually ranges from 20 to 40. Historically, removal of these lymph nodes (in an operation called axillary lymph node dissection, or ALND) was done for two reasons: to help stage breast cancer and to help prevent a regional recurrence of the disease. (Regional recurrence of breast cancer occurs when breast cancer cells that have migrated to nearby lymph nodes give rise to a new tumor.)

Because removing multiple lymph nodes at the same time has been associated with adverse effects, the possibility that SLNB alone might be sufficient for staging breast cancer in women who have no clinical signs of axillary lymph node metastasis, such as swollen or "matted" (clumped or stuck together) nodes, was investigated.

In a phase III trial involving 5,611 women with breast cancer and no clinical signs of axillary metastasis, researchers from the National Surgical Adjuvant Breast and Bowel Project, which is a National Cancer Institute (NCI) clinical trials cooperative group, randomly assigned participants to receive SLNB alone or SLNB plus ALND. The women in the two groups whose sentinel lymph node(s) were negative for cancer (a total of 3,989 women) were then followed for an average of 8 years. Most of the women (87.5 percent) had a lumpectomy, and the rest had a mastectomy. Nearly 88 percent of the women also received adjuvant systemic therapy (chemotherapy, hormonal therapy, or both), and 82 percent had external-beam radiation therapy to the affected breast.

The researchers found no differences in overall survival and disease-free survival between the two groups of women. Based on these results, it was concluded that ALND might not be necessary for women with clinically negative axillary lymph nodes and a negative SLNB whose breast cancer is treated with surgery, adjuvant systemic therapy, and external-beam radiation therapy.

Subsequently, the American College of Surgeons Oncology Group, which is another NCI clinical trials cooperative group, reported findings from an additional phase III clinical trial, this one testing whether women with a positive sentinel lymph node but no clinical evidence of axillary lymph node metastasis could be safely treated with tumor removal and no further lymph node surgery other than the SLNB. In this trial, 891 women were randomly assigned to SLNB only or ALND after SLNB. All of the women were treated with lumpectomy. More than 95 percent of them also received adjuvant systemic therapy (chemotherapy, hormone therapy, or both), and about 90 percent received external-beam radiation therapy to the affected breast.

When the results of this trial were reported, the patients had been followed for a median of 6.3 years. The two groups of women had similar 5-year overall survival (92.5 percent in the SLNB-only group versus 91.8 percent in the SLNB plus ALND group) and 5-year disease-free survival (83.9 percent in the SLNB-only group and 82.2 percent in the SLNB plus ALND group). The researchers concluded that SLNB alone is safe and does not affect the survival of women who have sentinel lymph node metastasis but no clinical signs of other lymph node involvement and whose breast cancer is treated with surgery, systemic therapy, and external-beam radiation therapy. The excellent outcome in this trial for women treated with SLNB without ALND is likely due, at least in part, to the ability of local radiation therapy and modern systemic treatments to effectively treat breast cancer cells that may have spread to other axillary lymph nodes besides the sentinel node or to other parts of the body.

What has research shown about the use of SLNB in melanoma?

Researchers have investigated whether patients with melanoma whose sentinel lymph node is negative for cancer and who have no clinical signs of other lymph node involvement can also be spared more extensive lymph node surgery at the time of primary tumor removal. A meta-analysis of 71 studies that involved data from 25,240 patients suggests that the answer to this question is "yes." This meta-analysis found that the risk of regional lymph node recurrence in patients with a negative SLNB was 5 percent or less.

Another question posed by researchers is whether SLNB plus the removal of the remaining regional lymph nodes (called completion lymph node dissection, or CLND) if the sentinel lymph node is positive for cancer has a therapeutic benefit for melanoma patients in terms of disease-free survival and melanoma-specific survival (length of time until death from melanoma). To address this question, NCI, the National Institutes of Health, and the John Wayne Cancer Institute are sponsoring a large phase III clinical trial called the Multicenter Selective Lymphadenectomy Trial II, or MSLT-II. In this trial, more than 1,900 patients with positive sentinel lymph nodes but no clinical evidence of other lymph node involvement are being randomly assigned to immediate CLND or regular ultrasound examination of the remaining regional lymph nodes and CLND if signs of additional lymph node metastasis appear. The patients in this trial will be followed for 10 years.

Chapter 10: Prostate-Specific Antigen (PSA) Test

- The PSA test measures the blood level of PSA, a protein that is produced by the prostate gland. The higher a man's PSA level, the more likely it is that he has prostate cancer. However, there are additional reasons for having an elevated PSA level, and some men who have prostate cancer do not have elevated PSA.

- The PSA test has been widely used to screen men for prostate cancer. It is also used to monitor men who have been diagnosed with prostate cancer to see if their cancer has recurred (come back) after initial treatment or is responding to therapy.

- Some advisory groups now recommend against the use of the PSA test to screen for prostate cancer because the benefits, if any, are small and the harms can be substantial. None recommend its use without a detailed discussion of the pros and cons of using the test.

What is the PSA test?

Prostate-specific antigen, or PSA, is a protein produced by cells of the prostate gland. The PSA test measures the level of PSA in a man's blood. For this test, a blood sample is sent to a laboratory for analysis. The results are usually reported as nanograms of PSA per milliliter (ng/mL) of blood.

The blood level of PSA is often elevated in men with prostate cancer, and the PSA test was originally approved by the FDA in 1986 to monitor the progression of prostate cancer in men who had already been diagnosed with the disease. In 1994, the FDA approved the use of the PSA test in conjunction with a digital rectal exam (DRE) to test asymptomatic men for prostate cancer. Men who report prostate symptoms often undergo PSA testing (along with a DRE) to help doctors determine the nature of the problem.

In addition to prostate cancer, a number of benign (not cancerous) conditions can cause a man's PSA level to rise. The most frequent benign prostate conditions that cause an elevation in PSA level are prostatitis (inflammation of the prostate) and benign prostatic hyperplasia (BPH) (enlargement of the prostate). There is no evidence that prostatitis or BPH leads to prostate cancer, but it is possible for a man to have one or both of these conditions and to develop prostate cancer as well.

Is the PSA test recommended for prostate cancer screening?

Until recently, many doctors and professional organizations encouraged yearly PSA screening for men beginning at age 50. Some organizations recommended that men who are at higher risk of prostate cancer, including African American men and men whose father or brother had prostate cancer, begin screening at age 40 or 45. However, as more has been learned about both the benefits and harms of prostate cancer screening, a number of organizations have begun to caution against routine population screening. Although some organizations continue to recommend PSA screening, there is widespread agreement that any man who is considering getting tested should first be informed in detail about the potential harms and benefits.

Currently, Medicare provides coverage for an annual PSA test for all Medicare-eligible men age 50 and older. Many private insurers cover PSA screening as well.

What is a normal PSA test result?

There is no specific normal or abnormal level of PSA in the blood. In the past, most doctors considered PSA levels of 4.0 ng/mL and lower as normal. Therefore, if a man had a PSA level above 4.0 ng/mL, doctors would often recommend a prostate biopsy to determine whether prostate cancer was present.

However, more recent studies have shown that some men with PSA levels below 4.0 ng/mL have prostate cancer and that many men with higher levels do not have prostate cancer. In addition, various factors can cause a man's PSA level to fluctuate. For example, a man's PSA level often rises if he has prostatitis or a urinary tract infection. Prostate biopsies and prostate surgery also increase PSA level. Conversely, some drugs—including finasteride and dutasteride, which are used to treat BPH—lower a man's PSA level. PSA level may also vary somewhat across testing laboratories.

Another complicating factor is that studies to establish the normal range of PSA levels have been conducted primarily in populations of white men. Although expert opinions vary, there is no clear consensus regarding the optimal PSA threshold for recommending a prostate biopsy for men of any racial or ethnic group.

In general, however, the higher a man's PSA level, the more likely it is that he has prostate cancer. Moreover, continuous rise in a man's PSA level over time may also be a sign of prostate cancer.

What if a screening test shows an elevated PSA level?

If a man who has no symptoms of prostate cancer chooses to undergo prostate cancer screening and is found to have an elevated PSA level, the doctor may recommend another PSA test to confirm the original finding. If the PSA level is still high, the doctor may recommend that the man continue with PSA tests and DREs at regular intervals to watch for any changes over time.

If a man's PSA level continues to rise or if a suspicious lump is detected during a DRE, the doctor may recommend additional tests to determine the nature of the problem. A urine test may be recommended to check for a urinary tract infection. The doctor may also recommend imaging tests, such as a transrectal ultrasound, x-rays, or cystoscopy.

If prostate cancer is suspected, the doctor will recommend a prostate biopsy. During this procedure, multiple samples of prostate tissue are collected by inserting hollow needles into the prostate and then withdrawing them. Most often, the needles are inserted through the wall of the rectum (transrectal biopsy); however, the needles may also be inserted through the skin between the scrotum and the anus (transperineal biopsy). A pathologist then examines the collected tissue under a microscope. The doctor may use ultrasound to view the prostate during the biopsy, but ultrasound cannot be used alone to diagnose prostate cancer.

What are some of the limitations and potential harms of the PSA test for prostate cancer screening?

Detecting prostate cancer early may not reduce the chance of dying from prostate cancer. When used in screening, the PSA test can help detect small tumors that do not cause symptoms. Finding a small tumor, however, may not necessarily reduce a man's chance of dying from prostate cancer. Some tumors found through PSA testing grow so slowly that they are unlikely to threaten a man's life. Detecting tumors that are not life threatening is called "overdiagnosis," and treating these tumors is called "overtreatment."

Overtreatment exposes men unnecessarily to the potential complications and harmful side effects of treatments for early prostate cancer, including surgery and radiation therapy. The side effects of these treatments include urinary incontinence (inability to control urine flow), problems with bowel function, erectile dysfunction (loss of erections, or having erections that are inadequate for sexual intercourse), and infection.

In addition, finding cancer early may not help a man who has a fast-growing or aggressive tumor that may have spread to other parts of the body before being detected.

The PSA test may give false-positive or false-negative results. A false-positive test result occurs when a man's PSA level is elevated but no cancer is actually present. A false-positive test result may create anxiety for a man and his family and lead to additional medical procedures, such as a prostate biopsy, that can be harmful. Possible side effects of biopsies include serious infections, pain, and bleeding.

Most men with an elevated PSA level turn out not to have prostate cancer; only about 25 percent of men who have a prostate biopsy due to an elevated PSA level actually have prostate cancer.

A false-negative test result occurs when a man's PSA level is low even though he actually has prostate cancer. False-negative test results may give a man, his family, and his doctor false assurance that he does not have cancer, when he may in fact have a cancer that requires treatment.

What research has been done to study prostate cancer screening?

Several randomized trials of prostate cancer screening have been carried out. One of the largest is the Prostate, Lung,

Colorectal, and Ovarian (PLCO) Cancer Screening Trial, which NCI conducted to determine whether certain screening tests can help reduce the numbers of deaths from several common cancers. In the prostate portion of the trial, the PSA test and DRE were evaluated for their ability to decrease a man's chances of dying from prostate cancer.

The PLCO investigators found that men who underwent annual prostate cancer screening had a higher incidence of prostate cancer than men in the control group but the same rate of deaths from the disease. Overall, the results suggest that many men were treated for prostate cancers that would not have been detected in their lifetime without screening. Consequently, these men were exposed unnecessarily to the potential harms of treatment.

A second large trial, the European Randomized Study of Screening for Prostate Cancer (ERSPC), compared prostate cancer deaths in men randomly assigned to PSA-based screening or no screening. As in the PLCO, men in ERSPC who were screened for prostate cancer had a higher incidence of the disease than control men. In contrast to the PLCO, however, men who were screened had a lower rate of death from prostate cancer.

The United States Preventive Services Task Force has analyzed the data from the PLCO, ERSPC, and other trials and estimated that, for every 1,000 men ages 55 to 69 years who are screened every 1 to 4 years for a decade:

- 0 to 1 death from prostate cancer would be avoided.

- 100 to 120 men would have a false-positive test result that leads to a biopsy, and about one-third of the men who get a biopsy would experience at least moderately bothersome symptoms from the biopsy.

- 110 men would be diagnosed with prostate cancer. About 50 of these men would have a complication from treatment, including erectile dysfunction in 29 men, urinary incontinence in 18 men, serious cardiovascular events in 2 men, deep vein thrombosis or pulmonary embolism in 1 man, and death due to the treatment in less than 1 man.

How is the PSA test used in men who have been treated for prostate cancer?

The PSA test is used to monitor patients who have a history of prostate cancer to see if their cancer has recurred (come back). If a man's PSA level begins to rise after prostate cancer treatment, it may be the first sign of a recurrence.

Such a "biochemical relapse" typically appears months or years before other clinical signs and symptoms of prostate cancer recurrence.

However, a single elevated PSA measurement in a patient who has a history of prostate cancer does not always mean that the cancer has come back. A man who has been treated for prostate cancer should discuss an elevated PSA level with his doctor. The doctor may recommend repeating the PSA test or performing other tests to check for evidence of a recurrence. The doctor may look for a trend of rising PSA level over time rather than a single elevated PSA level.

What does an increase in PSA level mean for a man who has been treated for prostate cancer?

If a man's PSA level rises after prostate cancer treatment, his doctor will consider a number of factors before recommending further treatment. Additional treatment based on a single PSA test is not recommended. Instead, a rising trend in PSA level over time in combination with other findings, such as an abnormal result on imaging tests, may lead a man's doctor to recommend further treatment.

How are researchers trying to improve the PSA test?

Scientists are investigating ways to improve the PSA test to give doctors the ability to better distinguish cancerous from benign conditions and slow-growing cancers from fast-growing, potentially lethal cancers. Some of the methods being studied include:

- *Free versus total PSA.* The amount of PSA in the blood that is "free" (not bound to other proteins) divided by the total amount of PSA (free plus bound). Some evidence suggests that a lower proportion of free PSA may be associated with more aggressive cancer.

- *PSA density of the transition zone.* The blood level of PSA divided by the volume of the transition zone of the prostate. The transition zone is the interior part of the prostate that surrounds the urethra. Some evidence suggests that this measure may be more accurate at detecting prostate cancer than the standard PSA test.

- *Age-specific PSA reference ranges.* Because a man's PSA level tends to increase with age, it has been suggested that the use of age-specific PSA reference ranges may increase the accuracy of PSA tests. However, age-specific reference ranges have not been generally favored because their use may delay the detection of prostate cancer in many men.

- *PSA velocity and PSA doubling time.* PSA velocity is the rate of change in a man's PSA level over time, expressed as ng/mL per year. PSA doubling time is the period of time over which a man's PSA level doubles. Some evidence suggests that the rate of increase in a man's PSA level may be helpful in predicting whether he has prostate cancer.

- *Pro-PSA.* Pro-PSA refers to several different inactive precursors of PSA. There is some evidence that pro-PSA is more strongly associated with prostate cancer than with BPH. One recently approved test combines measurement of a form of pro-PSA called [-2]proPSA with measurements of PSA and free PSA. The resulting "prostate health index" can be used to help a man with a PSA level of between 4 and 10 ng/mL decide whether he should have a biopsy.

Chapter 11: Tests to Detect Colorectal Cancer and Polyps

- Colorectal cancer is a disease in which cells in the colon or rectum become abnormal and divide without control, forming a mass called a tumor.
- The exact causes of colorectal cancer are not known. However, studies show that certain factors increase a person's chance of developing colorectal cancer.
- Health care providers may suggest one or more tests for colorectal cancer screening, including a fecal occult blood test (FOBT); sigmoidoscopy; regular, or standard, colonoscopy; virtual colonoscopy; or double contrast barium enema (DCBE).
- People should talk with their health care provider about when to begin screening for colorectal cancer, what tests to have, the benefits and risks (potential harms) of each test, and how often to schedule appointments.
- New methods, such as the genetic testing of stool samples, to screen for colorectal cancer are under study.

What is colorectal cancer?

Colorectal cancer is a disease in which cells in the colon or rectum become abnormal and divide without control, forming a mass called a tumor. (The colon and rectum are parts of the body's digestive system, which takes up nutrients from food and water, and stores solid waste until it passes out of the body.)

Colorectal cancer cells may also invade and destroy the tissue around them. In addition, they may break away from the tumor and spread to form new tumors in other parts of the body.

Colorectal cancer is the third most common type of non-skin cancer in men (after prostate cancer and lung cancer) and in women (after breast cancer and lung cancer). It is the second leading cause of cancer death in the United States after lung cancer. Although the rate of new colorectal cancer cases and deaths is decreasing in this country, an estimated 141,210 new cases of colorectal cancer and 49,380 deaths from this disease are expected to occur in 2011.

Who is at risk of developing colorectal cancer?

The exact causes of colorectal cancer are not known. However, studies have shown that certain factors are linked to an increased chance of developing this disease, including the following:

- *Age*—Colorectal cancer is more likely to occur as people get older. Although this disease can occur at any age, most people who develop colorectal cancer are over age 50.

- *Polyps*—Polyps are abnormal growths that protrude from the inner wall of the colon or rectum. They are relatively common in people over age 50. Most polyps are benign (noncancerous), but experts believe that the majority of colorectal cancers develop in polyps known as adenomas. Detecting and removing these growths may help prevent colorectal cancer. The procedure to remove polyps is called a polypectomy.

  Some individuals may be genetically predisposed to develop polyps. Familial adenomatous polyposis, or FAP, is a rare, inherited condition in which hundreds of polyps develop in the colon and rectum. Because individuals with this condition are extremely likely to develop colorectal cancer, they are often treated with surgery to remove the colon and rectum in an operation called a colectomy. Rectum-sparing surgery may also be an option. In addition, the Food and Drug Administration (FDA) has approved an anti-inflammatory drug, celecoxib, for the treatment of FAP. Doctors may prescribe this drug in combination with surveillance and surgery to manage FAP.

- *Personal history*—A person who has already had colorectal cancer is at an increased risk of developing colorectal cancer a second time. Also, research studies have shown that some women with a history of ovarian, uterine, or breast cancer have a higher than average chance of developing colorectal cancer.

- *Family history*—Close relatives (parents, siblings, or children) of a person who has had colorectal cancer are somewhat more likely to develop this type of cancer themselves, especially if the family member developed the cancer at a young age. If many family members have had colorectal cancer, the chances increase even more.

- *Ulcerative colitis or Crohn colitis*—Ulcerative colitis is a condition that causes inflammation and sores (ulcers) in the lining of the colon. Crohn colitis (also called Crohn disease) causes chronic inflammation of the gastrointestinal tract, most often of the small intestine (the part of the digestive tract that is located between the stomach and the large intestine). People who have ulcerative colitis or Crohn colitis may be more likely to develop colorectal cancer than people who do not have these conditions.

- *Diet*—Some evidence suggests that the development of colorectal cancer may be associated with high dietary consumption of red and processed meats and low consumption of whole grains, fruits, and vegetables. Researchers are exploring what role these and other dietary components play in the development of colorectal cancer.

- *Exercise*—Some evidence suggests that a sedentary lifestyle may be associated with an increased risk of developing colorectal cancer. In contrast, people who exercise regularly may have a decreased risk of developing colorectal cancer.

- *Smoking*—Increasing evidence from epidemiologic studies suggests that cigarette smoking, particularly long-term smoking, increases the risk of colorectal cancer.

What is screening, and why is it important?

Screening is checking for health problems before they cause symptoms. Colorectal cancer screening can detect cancer; polyps; nonpolypoid lesions, which are flat or slightly depressed areas of abnormal cell growth; and other conditions. Nonpolypoid lesions occur less often than polyps, but they can also develop into colorectal cancer.

If colorectal cancer screening reveals a problem, diagnosis and treatment can occur promptly. In addition, finding and removing polyps or other areas of abnormal cell growth may be one of the most effective ways to prevent colorectal cancer development. Also, colorectal cancer is generally more treatable when it is found early, before it has had a chance to spread.

What methods are used to screen people for colorectal cancer?

Health care providers may suggest one or more of the following tests for colorectal cancer screening:

- *Fecal occult blood test (FOBT)*—This test checks for hidden blood in fecal material (stool).

Currently, two types of FOBT are available. One type, called guaiac FOBT, uses the chemical guaiac to detect heme in samples of stool. Heme is the iron-containing component of the blood protein hemoglobin. Usually, samples of stool from three different bowel movements are collected for guaiac FOBT. The other type of FOBT, called immunochemical (or immunohistochemical) FOBT, uses antibodies to detect human hemoglobin protein in samples of stool. Depending on the type of immunochemical FOBT, stool samples from one to three bowel movements are collected. Studies have shown that FOBT, when performed every 1 to 2 years in people ages 50 to 80, can help reduce the number of deaths due to colorectal cancer by 15 to 33 percent.

- *Sigmoidoscopy*—In this test, the rectum and lower colon are examined using a lighted instrument called a sigmoidoscope. During sigmoidoscopy, precancerous and cancerous growths in the rectum and lower colon can be found and either removed or biopsied. Studies suggest that regular screening with sigmoidoscopy after age 50 can help reduce the number of deaths from colorectal cancer. A thorough cleansing of the lower colon is necessary for this test.

- *Colonoscopy*—In this test, the rectum and entire colon are examined using a lighted instrument called a colonoscope. During colonoscopy, precancerous and cancerous growths throughout the colon can be found and either removed or biopsied, including growths in the upper part of the colon, where they would be missed by sigmoidoscopy. However, it is not yet known for certain whether colonoscopy can help reduce the number of deaths from colorectal cancer. A thorough cleansing of the colon is necessary before this test, and most patients receive some form of sedation.

- *Virtual colonoscopy (also called computerized tomographic colonography)*—In this test, special x-ray equipment is used to produce pictures of the colon and rectum. A computer then assembles these pictures into detailed images that can show polyps and other abnormalities. Because it is less invasive than standard colonoscopy and sedation is not needed, virtual colonoscopy may cause less discomfort and take less time to perform. As with standard colonoscopy, a thorough cleansing of the colon is necessary before this test. Whether virtual colonoscopy can reduce the number of deaths from colorectal cancer is not yet known.

- *Double contrast barium enema (DCBE)*—In this test, a series of x-rays of the entire colon and rectum are taken after the patient is given an enema with a barium solution and air is introduced into the colon. The barium and air help to outline the colon and rectum on the x-rays. Research shows that DCBE may miss small polyps. It detects about 30 to 50 percent of the cancers that can be found with standard colonoscopy.

In addition, doctors often perform a digital rectal exam (DRE) during routine physical examinations and may use this test to check for abnormal areas in the lower part of the rectum. They may also perform a single-specimen guaiac FOBT on stool collected during a DRE, but research has shown that this approach is not very accurate and cannot be recommended as the only method of screening for colorectal cancer.

Scientists are still studying colorectal cancer screening methods, both alone and in combination, to determine how effective they are. Studies are also under way to clarify the potential risks, or harms, of each screening test.

How can people and their health care providers decide which colorectal cancer screening test(s) to use and how often to be screened?

Several major organizations, including the U.S. Preventive Services Task Force (a group of experts convened by the U.S. Public Health Service), the American Cancer Society, and professional societies, have developed guidelines for colorectal cancer screening. Although some details of their recommendations vary regarding which screening tests to use and how often to be screened, all of these organizations support screening for colorectal cancer.

People should talk with their health care provider about when to begin screening for colorectal cancer, what tests to have, the benefits and harms of each test, and how often to schedule appointments.

The decision to have a certain test will take into account several factors, including the following:

- The person's age, medical history, family history, and general health

- The accuracy of the test
- The potential harms of the test
- The preparation required for the test
- Whether sedation is necessary during the test
- The follow-up care after the test
- The convenience of the test
- The cost of the test and the availability of insurance coverage

The following list outlines some of the advantages and disadvantages, including potential harms, of the colorectal cancer screening tests.

<u>Fecal Occult Blood Test (FOBT)</u>

- *Advantages*:
    - No cleansing of the colon is necessary.
    - Samples can be collected at home.
    - Cost is low compared with other colorectal cancer screening tests.
    - Does not cause bleeding or tearing/perforation of the lining of the colon.
- *Disadvantages*:
    - Fails to detect most polyps and some cancers.

- False-positive results (the test suggests an abnormality when none is present) are possible.
- Dietary restrictions may be needed before the test.
- Additional procedures, such as colonoscopy, may be needed if FOBT indicates an abnormality.

Sigmoidoscopy

- *Advantages*:
  - Test is usually quick, with few complications.
  - For most patients, discomfort is minimal.
  - In some cases, the doctor may be able to perform a biopsy and remove polyps during the test, if necessary.
  - Less extensive cleansing of the colon is necessary for this test than for a colonoscopy.

- *Disadvantages*:
  - Any polyps in the upper part of the colon will be missed because the test allows the doctor to view only the rectum and the lower part of the colon.

- o Very small risk of bleeding or tearing/perforation of the lining of the colon.
- o Additional procedures, such as colonoscopy, may be needed if the test indicates an abnormality.

Colonoscopy

- *Advantages*:
  - o Allows the doctor to view the rectum and the entire colon.
  - o Doctor can perform a biopsy and remove polyps or other abnormal tissue during the test, if necessary.
- *Disadvantages*:
  - o May not detect all small polyps, nonpolypoid lesions, and cancers, but is one of the most sensitive tests currently available.
  - o Thorough cleansing of the colon is necessary before this test.
  - o Some form of sedation is used in most cases.

- o Although uncommon, complications such as bleeding and/or tearing/perforation of the lining of the colon can occur.

Virtual Colonoscopy

- *Advantages*:
  - o Allows the doctor to view the rectum and the entire colon.
  - o No risk of bleeding or tearing/perforation of the lining of the colon.
- *Disadvantages*:
  - o May not detect all small polyps, nonpolypoid lesions, and cancers.
  - o Thorough cleansing of the colon is necessary before the test.
  - o If a polyp or nonpolypoid lesion 6 to 9 millimeters in size or larger is detected, standard colonoscopy, usually immediately after the virtual procedure, will be recommended to remove the polyp or lesion or perform a biopsy.

Double-Contrast Barium Enema (DCBE)

- *Advantages*:
  - o Usually allows the doctor to view the rectum and the entire colon.

- o Complications are rare.
- o No sedation is needed.
- • *Disadvantages*:
  - o May not detect some small polyps and cancers.
  - o Thorough cleansing of the colon is necessary before the test.
  - o False-positive results are possible.
  - o Doctor cannot perform a biopsy or remove polyps during the test.
  - o Additional procedures are necessary if the test indicates an abnormality.

Do insurance companies pay for colorectal cancer screening?

People should check with their health insurance provider to determine their colorectal cancer screening benefits. Because virtual colonoscopy is a fairly new procedure, reimbursement policies may be more uncertain than for other types of screening. Medicare covers several colorectal cancer screening tests for its beneficiaries.

What happens if a colorectal cancer screening test shows an abnormality?

If a screening test finds an abnormality, the health care provider will perform a physical exam and evaluate the person's personal and family medical history. Additional tests may be ordered. These tests may include x-rays of the gastrointestinal tract, sigmoidoscopy, or, most often, colonoscopy (see Question 4). The health care provider may also order a blood test called a CEA assay to measure carcinoembryonic antigen, a protein that is sometimes detected in greater amounts in patients with colorectal cancer. If an abnormality is found during a sigmoidoscopy, a biopsy or polypectomy may be performed during the test, and a colonoscopy may be recommended. If an abnormality is found during a standard colonoscopy, a biopsy or polypectomy is performed to determine whether cancer is present. If an abnormality is detected during virtual colonoscopy, most patients would be referred for a standard colonoscopy the same day.

Are new tests under study for colorectal cancer screening?

Genetic testing of stool samples is being studied as a possible way to screen for colorectal cancer. The lining of the colon is constantly shedding cells into the stool. Testing stool samples for genetic alterations that occur in colorectal cancer cells may help doctors find evidence of cancer or precancerous growths. Research conducted thus far has shown that this kind of test can detect colorectal cancer in people already diagnosed with this disease by other means. However, more studies are needed to determine whether this type of test can accurately detect colorectal cancer or precancerous polyps in people who do not have symptoms.

Other MedicalCenter.com Publications

The Key Facts on Arthritis

The Key Facts on Breast Cancer

The Key Facts on Medicare

The Key Facts on Alzheimer's Disease

The Key Facts on Caring For Someone With

Alzheimer's Disease

The Key Facts on Cancer Series

All Titles Can Be Found at

www.Amazon.com

www.MedicalCenter.com